Don't Forget You

Simple Steps To Care For Your Well-Being

Dedication

I dedicate this booklet to my uncle for encouraging me to take action. And to my mom for always encouraging me to care for myself. I wouldn't be where I am without you. Thank you.

This book is for informational purposes only. It can not diagnose or prescribe treatment for any condition. If you need medical or mental health services, seek help from a licensed professional.

Table of Contents

Get more resources to help you care
for your well-being at:
NickMaizy.com/DFUbonus

caring for your well-being

"If you feel "burnout" setting in, if you feel demoralized and exhausted, it is best, for the sake of everyone, to withdraw and restore yourself." - Dalai Lama

Intentionally doing what you need for your well-being is self-care. It is caring for your mental and physical needs so you can be your best. It takes time, energy, a little planning, and being deliberate with what you do. You can do it and experience the amazing benefits of it.

Self-care is not selfish. We need to address this point. Caring for yourself is NOT selfish at all. Anyone at the top of their game, performing at a peak level, takes time to care for themselves so they can be at their best. You should too. It will help you be better for yourself and for those you care about.

Why is it so important now?

Self-care needs to be a priority. Don't put off doing it until things improve, you have more time available or you get caught up on your to do lists. You won't ever do it if you keep putting it off. Self-care is helpful when times are good and everything is going your way. But, that's not why I wrote this book. This book is here to make sure you care for yourself when times are not so good. You need to practice self-care even in the middle of a crisis. When you're scrambling to get everything done, you're falling behind, getting overwhelmed, and things are falling apart, you'll need it more than ever. Self-care is critical when things are not going your way. It's far too easy to put off caring for yourself when you need it the most.

Really that important?

You don't have to care for yourself if you don't want to. Nobody will make you. You may choose to allow the stress to mount, ignoring the needs of your mind and body.

Imagine for a minute you have a car that needs basic maintenance. You spent your hard earned money on that car and expect it to perform well and serve you the best that it can. The car needs an oil change. The junk in the engine is building up. You know you're supposed to change the oil, but you put it off because it is still running. Time continues to pass. You keep driving the car and don't pay attention to what it needs. Before long the tires get old too. Their tread wears down and they don't grip the road quite as well as they used to. If you continue to use that vehicle without caring for its needs, what will happen? I don't know exactly what will happen, but it will probably be awful. The engine may seize up and completely stop working. Or, you may crash because the tires didn't grip the road enough. All because you didn't take a little time and address what the car needed.

A little self-care for you is the maintenance for your car. If you don't do it immediately, you may not notice a difference. But, over time, the effects of neglecting self-care becomes more and more clear. Eventually, there will be negative consequences and they may keep you from experiencing the life you want. You can take small steps regularly to address stress, help you think clearer, and allow your body to perform better. I believe self-care should be a top priority in your life because anything worth doing requires your mind and/or body. Self-care will allow your mind and body to serve you the best that it can. It can also make life more enjoyable and help prevent burnout.

If you're worried that caring for yourself will in some way take away from others, then please listen carefully. Self-care allows you to be your best for yourself and for others. And a lack of self-care can compromise your health and limit your ability to serve others well. When you care for yourself, everyone wins!

Just Like You, Self-Care Is Unique

Each one of us is unique and has specific needs. The specific ways you can care for yourself may be a little different from the specific way I do. However, the similarities are greater than the differences. For example, some people need a little more or less sleep than others. Quality sleep benefits us all, though. Here we'll explore some general things that you can do for self-care. Then, you can adapt what you need for your specific needs, situation, and life to get the benefits you want.

You Need Your Body

The state of your body has an enormous impact on your entire life and it's the only one you get. You're stuck with it for the rest of your life. So, you need to take care of it. The better you care for it, the better it can care for you. There are simple things you can do that will help your body help you. They will take some work and require you to make the conscious choice to care for yourself. Remember, it's worth the effort and you will experience countless benefits.

The key ideas we'll explore are that it's good to move your body, put healthy things into it, allow it to rest, and get fresh air.

Move

Moving your body is good for it. Yes, your body is unique and specific exercises may benefit it more than others. You may already know some specific exercises that work well for your body. Perhaps they may not be the ones you enjoy the most. We will talk about doing specific things that you enjoy later. Right here, think of a few simple ways you can move your body more. Consider going for a walk, run, do some stretching, or lift some weights. Having a list of things you can do makes it easier to do them.

Don't have the energy to exercise? The funny little secret about exercising is it uses energy while it creates more energy. I know it sounds crazy, but it happens. Attempt to do good things for your body even when you don't feel like it. You will still reap the benefits. You can have progress or excuses. But, you can't have both.

Can I tell you another funny little secret? Most of the time I don't feel like exercising at all. What?!? How can I suggest that you do something that I don't want to do? Simple. I do what I need to do for my body even when I don't feel like it. Doing what you feel like doing typically won't get you what you want in the long-term. Get a little exercise, movement, or stretching.

Now, I will tell you another little secret. Sometimes the motivation starts after you do. I normally get motivated to exercise about 5-10 mins after I start. That's when I feel good and proud of myself for exercising. Yes, it would be great if the motivation came before I started. That would make things so much easier. Fortunately for us, we do not need motivation to start. Just start. Even a little exercise is great for the body and can help it handle stress, increase energy, and improve your overall health. If you want to care for yourself, then get some exercise regularly.

Nutrition

There are more diets out there than I want to count. I will not begin to tell you which is the best for you. Your body is unique and I'm not a dietician. I can say fuel your body with quality food and nutrition. If you want it to treat you well then, you need to treat it well. Honestly, I love the way a greasy burger and fries taste. But, they are crappy fuel for my body. And viewing food as fuel helps me to make the better choice for my health, body, and life. A monumental part of caring for yourself is choosing what you put into your body. I believe making a simple choice to eat real food (not processed), drink plenty of straight water, and limit sugar is a superb place to start. Your specifics may differ.

You may love processed sugary carbs washed down with a soda. It may be difficult to make the shift to a healthier diet. You don't have to change everything all at once. Even slight changes lead to benefits. All you have to do is start somewhere.

Rest

We all need sleep. Some people need a little more, some a little less. Sleep is essential for all of us. Fortunately, there are some brilliant and simple suggestions available requiring minimal effort that can lead to a more restful night's sleep.

Screens Off

Give yourself a 30 minute break from any screens before bed. The blue light emitted from electronic screens can affect your ability to get quality sleep. If you can't stay away from the screen, your device may have a built-in blue light filter you can turn on in the settings. Some people use special glasses that filter out the blue light.

Lights Out

Limiting the amount of light where you sleep can also help. This may include closing the blinds, turning off the T.V., or removing electronic devices that have little lights on them from the room.

Bedtime Routine

Routines are pretty much habits. The routine can be simple and still be powerful. Developing a simple routine to prepare yourself for bed can help your mind and body be ready to sleep. Brushing your teeth and preparing for the next day are just a few things you can build into your evening routine. Your routine should also include timing. Going to bed and getting up at the same time every day can aid in falling asleep and waking easier at your desired time.

Your Actions Count

What you do is important. It's crucial to understand that your actions affect your health. Your large actions can affect your health. Your small actions can affect your health too. Take a small step to caring for your body.

Get more resources to help you care for your one and only body at:
NickMaizy.com/DFUbonus

ADDRESS THE STRESS

"The day she let go of the things that were weighing her down, was the day she began to shine the brightest." - Katrina Mayer

There are many ways to define stress. The one I work from is that stress is when there is pressure or tension on a body. In today's world, it seems like we're always on the go. There are endless demands for our time and attention. Having too many demands and placed on us can lead to increased levels of stress. This may be why so many of us experience the effects of stress. You often hear people talking about stress as this evil, negative thing you have to fight against. That's not necessarily the case. If you feel stressed or notice some symptoms of stress, view that as information. That information can help you realize it may be time to do something different.

How Do You Feel Stress?

There are more different symptoms of stress than we can review here. How each one of us experiences the effects of stress varies as greatly as the ways we can care for ourselves. These are just a few. Noticing which one you experience can be a good thing. You can use that information as a suggestion your body and mind may need a little self-care.

Muscle Tension	On Edge/Anxious
Headaches	More Coffee/Alcohol
Irritability	Difficulty Deciding
Trouble Focusing	Changes in Eating
Resentment	Nervous Habits
Extra Sweating	Changes in Sleep

By being intentional, you can help your body address the stress to reduce its symptoms and can help you think clearer, have more energy, feel better and enjoy life more. Let's explore some simple ways you can reduce stress.

Breathing Exercises

Breathing techniques can be an amazing tool to help you reduce stress. You can calm the body and mind just by changing your breathing. While there are many variations of similar techniques here will look at just two.

Box/Square Breathing

Imagine a square with the number 4 on each side. The 4 represents how long you'll count for each part of the breath. To practice, find a quiet place where you can sit for a few minutes. You can sit on the ground or in a chair. Start by taking a few deep breaths in through the nose and out through the mouth. Then, when you're ready, gently close your eyes while exhaling. Breath in through your nose for a count of 4. Hold your breath for a count of 4. Exhale out your mouth for a count of 4. Inhale for a count of 4. And repeat.

Calming Breath

The calming breath technique is like box breathing, but with a different count. Once again, find a quiet place, sit, and take a few deep breaths. Gently close your eyes on while you exhale. This time breathe in through your nose for a count of 4, hold for a count of 7, and exhale through the mouth for a count of 8. And repeat.

Be Present

Being mentally present right where you're at can be a challenge. When you think about being somewhere else, it can rob the present moment from the power it has. Wishing to be somewhere other than where you're at right now can promote stress and steal any enjoyment you can have at the moment. Even when it's not the most pleasant moment, it can still be helpful to be mentally present. Wanting to do something different or be somewhere different will only reinforce that you're not where you want or doing what you want. This will focus your mental attention on what you're lacking and missing.

While in school, I learned about a fascinating study that has stuck with me ever since. The study focused on enjoyment and being mentally present. During the study participants had to drive in traffic, which is obviously not a pleasant task. They asked some participants to play music and try to distract themselves from the drive. They told the other participants to just drive without music or distractions. Then each group rated how enjoyable the drive was from 0 to 10. Interestingly, they found that the people who distracted themselves from the unpleasantness of traffic reported enjoying the trip less than those who were driving without being distracted.

While the study may not be earth shattering, it may have a lesson for us to learn. Living in the present moment offers benefits.

Mindfulness

Being fully present is not just about limiting distractions while driving. Mindfulness meditation is a practice of mentally being fully present. It can help calm the body and mind and reduce stress. If you're new to mindfulness or meditation, try it. Like most unfamiliar things, it can seem a little weird or different when you first start. Before long, it will become more natural and you'll experience the benefits faster. Especially when you're first starting mindfulness meditation, it helps to listen as someone guides you through the practice. It is more than just deep breathing with your eyes closed. There are many programs available to help you get started. Visit the resources below for some of my favorites or search for one that suits you. Starting and practicing is more important than picking the absolute best program.

Get To Nature

One very simple way to help reduce stress is to spend time in nature.

Getting outside with some fresh air and sunshine can help reduce stress. You could pair this with a little exercise by going for a walk in nature. The effect nature has on the body and mind is powerful. If you can't go for a long walk in nature every day, don't give up on this one. Some people have even found just adding a picture of nature on an office wall can help improve mood. So, get out in nature or at least enjoy viewing pictures of the great outdoors. It may help you relax.

Find more resources to help you address the stress at:
NickMaizy.com/DFUbonus

CHOOSE THE POSITIVE

"Things turn out best for the people who
make the best of the way things turn out."
- John Wooden

It's hard to stay positive when there are a lot of negative things going on around us. Even with all the things on the outside doesn't mean you have to let it negativity rein on the inside. Choosing to add something positive to your day can be a significant way to care for yourself. Can you make yourself be more positive? It's more than just saying out loud "will be more positive." It's what you do that counts.

Here are a few things you can do to help shift yourself to the positive.

Self-talk

Self-talk is the words you tell yourself. We all say things to ourselves. In fact, the most important words you'll hear are the ones you tell yourself. Would you want to hang around someone if they always said negative things to you, criticized you, and put you down? Would you? I know I wouldn't want to be around them. Nobody wants to be around that person. Often we say negative things to ourselves that we would never say to others. The point of positive self-talk is not stopping every single negative word or thought from entering your mind. It is being intentional with what you tell yourself.

The craziest thing about self-talk is that, over time, you'll believe the words you tell yourself. You can add positive words to your self-talk that encourage you and help you experience the life you want.

Ask "What would a friend say to encourage me right now?"

It may feel a little weird saying encouraging words to yourself at first. But, it is powerful, effective, worth the effort, and you'll get more comfortable with it after you practice. Try to encourage yourself out loud so you can hear the words. Again, I know it may be a little out of your comfort zone. Do it anyway. Giving yourself a pep talk can help you improve your mindset and take the steps you need to enjoy life more.

Focus

What you focus on grows. The more you focus on something, the more attention it will take up in your mind. Being intentional with where you place your focus can have a massive impact on your life. Your focus affects your thoughts, which impact your actions, which guide your life.

Where do you focus your attention?

Your mind may naturally see the challenges or what may go wrong. If it does, that's okay. You can still be intentional and direct your focus to what will help you. Shifting your focus to the positive can be challenging. You don't have to make a massive shift all at once. Taking minor steps to direct your focus to the positive can help you make progress.

Enjoy Life

You can attempt to enjoy what you're doing more. Don't discredit this suggestion even if it sounds dumb or trivial. There is power in making your mind up that no matter what you will make the most of where you're at and enjoy it as much as possible. Think about it. What if you focus on the positive aspects of a situation, focused on the good and the possibilities even when things aren't what you want? There are always things that I'd prefer to be different. And focusing on all those things will cause me misery while I stay stuck. Or, I can do my best in the situation, try to enjoy it, while I make progress toward something better. The latter is what I want for me and what I want for you.

Choose

You may not choose what goes on around you. However, you will choose what you do about it. Adding a bit of positivity can be a significant way to care for yourself when there is a lot of negativity. When things aren't going right, it's more important than ever to add more things that will help you. Make the choice to be more positive with your self-talk and where you put your focus.. Be intentional and try to enjoy the little things and minor moments more while you make the most of where you're at.

Find more resources to help you choose the positive at:
NickMaizy.com/DFUbonus

YOU CAN DO IT

"You can do what you have to do, and sometimes you can do it even better than you think you can." - Jimmy Carter

Life is not perfect, it never will be. No matter what, you can make the best of where you're at, though. Making the best of it does not mean to accept life as it is without trying to change it for the better. Be where you're at, enjoy all the good that you can in your current situation. Accept that life is not perfect. While helping you be the best version of you that you can be. Caring for yourself can be a significant way to help your life improve without trying to change everything around you.

You can't do it all. Trying to do everything can lead to stress and overwhelm, which will not help with self-care. Starting is the smallest that can make it easier to begin with and easier to maintain. Start with a small, simple step that seems right for you. Once you enjoy some benefits, you can add another step.

Just say you start by practicing some deep breathing or mindfulness exercises. You find that it helps you think clearer and relax a bit. Then, it may be easier for you to sleep better at night. After a while, you work on improving your sleep. Before long, you have a little more energy and are less overwhelmed. You use your newfound energy to exercise some.

You don't have to start by doing it all at once. You just need to start.

It's What You Do

It all comes down to what you do. You can't do it all. The wonderful news is you definitely can do something. I want to share with you something I learned from one of my favorite supervisors. He taught me the importance of taking action during uncertainty. There were always changes at that job. We never knew when a change in procedure would come or what it would be. This supervisor would say these simple words that make the most sense. He would say, "do something." Even with all the uncertainty that we worked in, it made the most sense for us to take action. If we did the next right thing, we always ended up better off than if we waited until we knew the exact perfect step.

You need not be perfect or know the perfect next step. Just do something for you and your life. That is a superb place to start. Take a small step to care for yourself. Make it a habit. And keep improving.

After you start, keep at it. Keep caring for yourself. The more you practice self-care, the more benefits you'll get. When you repeat your actions they can become habits. Developing habits around caring for yourself can help you be healthy, happy, and enjoy life.

You are important.
Take steps to care for yourself.
It's worth the effort.